Cancer: The Cause and Answer !

By Conor A. Murphy

Started on April The First, of 2016 at 7:15 PM.

Finished on :

Friday May The 13th of 2016 at 4:10 PM

May this book be a blessing to all who read it and may they delight in this life saving Knowledge, SHALOM !!!

Thanks to Yeshua (Hebrew For Jesus) and my mother (Eileen Murphy) for leading me into true health and healing. Plus understanding how the body works and function !!! Shout out to my Marvelous Grandmother (Kathleen Murphy) for listening to me and guiding me.

Table Of Contents

Chapter 1 : Intro .

To begin, for "legal reasons" I will must state: This book and what it contains will not cure all cancer. Everyone is different with different bodies and internal, different health, age and chemistry. For true health is a filament of mind, body and soul. However, the keys to health which is knowledge contained in this book. Can be used for great health and will give your body great health, rather or not you do have cancer. This is not take a pill and see results, or do this one thing a day and cure cancer. No. This is a health lifestyle. If you want to be healthy and cancer free. You got to live and breathe great health. For a healthy mind, do what is right, medicate on what is pure, just and noble and do what has to be done. You got to cut off toxicity in your life. Have a great mind set and less stressful life. Cut off toxic people as well. You cant help a sick person who doesn't want to be healed. Like that sick man in the bible who sat near the healing pool for thirty eight years making up excuses. What did Jesus tell him to do: **Get up** and walk, basically. If you want good health. **Get up** and do it. You want success ? **Get up** and do it. It happens, when you make it happen. This book will take care of the body, how it works, what causes cancer and how to WAGE WAR against it. For mind and soul you must get right with your maker for a true Shalom!

Chapter 2: What Is Cancer ?

Before we can go into the cure of cancer. We must first go into what is cancer. Like wise leaders who study information about their enemy before going to war. It is vital to know what cancer is, before we talk about defeating it. Cancer is caused by toxicity in body. Your digestive system is your sewage system.

Every day you take in toxins and expel them out (Sewage) .These toxins are pushed out of the body through your urine and waste. Just like a sewage facility, your body can become overfilled with toxins and this causes problems. Your kidneys and your liver are overflowed so the toxins go elsewhere. This is where we get an excessive grouping of toxicity. The body, which knows how to fix it self. Will deal with the excess of toxicity in multiple ways such as pushing it out through the skin which is where people get acne, eczema, diabetes and various other issues. They are not the root problem, they are signs of the internal problem going on inside. The inside coming out. If there is disorder and chaos on the inside, it will show up on the outside. Tumors form from these excess toxins, for the body takes the toxicity away from where it can damage vital organs into lymph nodes where they are stored. So the body can properly deport out the toxins when the digestive system is read to handle them. Some of this sewage comes from the cells, the body deports the sewage to the kidneys to be eliminated. The waste must be brought to the outside of the body for waste cannot stay in the body without harming it. When the kidneys, liver and digestive system are backed up and cannot process anymore waste. Then the toxins group together and form tumors and lymph nodes that build up and grow bigger and cancerous. That is why it is dangerous to cut one of those off. Because when you do, there is a chance that the toxicity will escape its confinement and spread to the nearby area, infecting and corrupting the nearby cells. This is a main cause of cancer rapidly spreading around the body. For specific cells do not travel like vagabonds. An ear cell has no business in the leg, it is not assigned to the leg and will not travel to the leg, but how does a corrupt, cancerous, infected ear cell go to the leg ? Through the blood stream toxins and free radicals that cause cancer spread around the body. They get into the blood system and ride it like a monorail express to seek and destroy your body !!! When cells are full of toxicity and surrounded by it. Then they themselves start to mutate. Now you have a rapid, fast growing cancer to deal with. NOT GOOD !!! Your body is natural, and was made to consume natural food. Artificial, manmade "gunge", like Glutens, pesticides and GMOS among other unnatural products are difficult for the body to process and break down, so they consume more time in the stomach and stay their longer versus natural food.

This is an epic, epidemic in society. GMOS and other cancerous toxins and chemicals are being put in food poisoning millions all across the world, especially in America. It's shameful, evil and blood money. It must end and we must return to natural food with natural ingredients for natural health for our natural bodies which God created. Natural Natural Natural.

Chapter 3 : Basic Chemistry

PH : is a numeric scale used to test/calculate the toxicity and acidity of things. The range goes from 0-14 with 7 being natural, below seven being acidic and above seven being alkaline. Most water has an PH of seven or slightly above. Your body being about 70% water should have a PH of seven or slightly above to have good health. A rusted up old car battery has a PH level of about 1 or less. Pig, beef, shellfish, alcohol and dairy products are some of the items that have a very acidic PH level. What items have a high alkaline PH level are: raw spinach, broccoli, celery to name a few. The PH level of your body play a huge role in your healthy. People who are acidic are more prone to sickness and disease. For their body is a great place for parasites, bad bacteria and cancer to grow and thrive in. For when the PH is down, the body has to work more to digest food, to defeat sicknesses and illnesses and keep the body in good health. It also makes breaking down and deportation of toxins and chemicals in the body, a harder and longer process to detox. The body is also run down by what is called the "SAD" diet. The "Standard American Diet" is full of high sugar processed food that take a toll on the body, stress it out and drain you of your minerals and vitamins in order to try and balance itself out in an over toxic environment that is fueled by a bad diet, little to no working out and not enough sleep and too much stress. Look at a bottle of coke a cola. All their cancerous ingredients, a bottle of coke poured on a car with erode away the paint and leave a mark. Do you want that going in your body ! Holding coke in your mouth would burn right through your jaw if your mouth didn't pump out alkaline water rapidly !   To have a good PH (about 7.35 to 8.50) is to have good health. In this world full of acidic foods we must eat proportionally about 80-70% good, healthy food and about 20-30% that is pleasure food. Chemo therapy has an extremely low PH: rating. More acidic than car batteries. No wonder it destroys the body and kills the hair. Who in their right mind believes that helps the body !!!

Chapter 4: Evil Chemo:

Chemo is deadly chemicals that evolved from mustard gas research in the 1940's-50's. It was tested on animals and people. It would sometimes decrease their tumors, but , BUT !!! It will kill them a short while after. This was amazing to the western health officials back then for this was their first time that they had used something synthetic that decreased tumors. Chemo drugs are very deadly that kill cells and corrupt their DNA causing mutations and free radicals. Doctors don't tell their patients that much. Most doctors will tell their patients very little, certainly won't tell their patients everything about chemo. They might say, oh you will lose your hair, may age quicker, lose your appetite and energy, they certainly don't tell them that chemo has an estimated average of a high 90% failure rating. Do you know why that is ???? Well when you pump highly toxic, lethal chemicals into the body. That cause your hair to fall out, and your skin to become aged and leathery. As you age quickly and disintegrate. Do you possibly think that chemo that causes this is good for you ??? HELL NO !!! Its evil, satanic and destructive to the body. Look at actors and celebrities who have taken chemo. They look terrible afterwards and lose themselves. Chemo drugs poison the cells in the body, not just the cancer cells. The doctors have no control over where the poison goes specifically in the body and what cells they corrupt. Extremely life threatening damage take place in the body after chemo. The toxins go through your liver, which we learned about in chapter 1, and clog the liver and kidneys damaging them both. Some patients have to wear dippers because they cannot control their bladder due to the drugs.

A lot of these toxins in the drugs are known carcinogens, and listed by the U.S national a toxicology department as "Cancer Causing Chemicals". So not only will chemo weaken your immune system, they will cause other cancers to grow in body. Defeating the purpose of "curing cancer". That is why, a lot of cancer patients have had the same story. They were diagnosed with cancer, had chemo therapy, the cancer/tumor died down or got smaller. People were happy. Then later on, the cancer returns, it has spread and it is more aggressive and worse than before. Do you know why ? It's because the so called "Doctors" are not dealing with the root cause. You got to pull the weeds out by their roots to stop them. Chopping them up, cutting them up and operating on them won't get rid of them. The doctors are treating the symptoms which is what they do in the majority and then recommend all these pills and treatments so they can make money off of you. Money off of your bad health. Because if people were all well and healthy. Then a lot of these doctors, big pharma companies and organizations would go out of business. Chemo and the pill business in general is a huge industry. +2 trillion $ BIG!!! Like I said before, this is blood money. Profiting off of peoples sickness and disease. In 2004 there was a ground breaking study "The Contribution of Cytotoxic Chemotherapy to 5-year Survival in Adult Malignancies" found that the overall contribution to five year survival is only on average a whopping 2% !!! Now some cancers did respond better to chemo than others. But did they find a cure ? No. This only showed that the patients lived five years with cancer. If they dropped dead after five years and one day, they would still have contributed to the percent. Scandalous !!! Same with radiation treatment. This is just pure ignorance. You don't treat the symptoms, you treat the cause. These doctors do not understand how the body works, nor the bacteria that lives inside of it. If your doctor says you have an "autoimmune" problem. They don't really know what you have because there is no such thing as an "autoimmune problem" !!! There is simply cause and effect. People can judge and say whatever they like but nature is ruled by chemistry and physics. By simple cause and effect. Yeshua (Jesus) called it "You reap what you sow" if people are going to live unhealthy and put junk/toxic food in their body then people will be unhealthy and their body will be junk and toxic. People are what they eat. If someone says "your/my diet doesn't affect you/me" then ask them why they won't eat/drink a bunch of poison. It the same concept. Whether poison on its own, or in the food. So if your body is toxic and acidic. Is it wise to use chemo to fix it ? Certainly not. Chemo is a hotter acid than the cancer acid toxins that are mutating the human cells. Whoever taught this was a great idea lacks understanding for how the body works. You cannot neutralize acid with more acids. Its basic chemistry that you suppress an acid with alkaline. Using acid with another acid, will only make more acid ! And because its acids that are destroying the tissue and you're going to add more acid. What are you doing ? You're not making it better, you're making it worse !!! Basic Chemistry. There is nothing new under the sun, what works, works, what doesn't, doesn't. If there is a chemo leak. People have to quarantine the area of impact and get in chemical and specialist. Because its not natural and is toxic. Also to be noted is that most cancer NOT ALL but most "Non Profit Cancer Organizations" where people donate money to "find a cure for cancer" and such. The money from those organizations mostly goes to the big pharmaceutical who produce more toxic pills, rarely does this money go to alternative forms of medicine.

Chapter 5 : Detoxify !!!

Cancer is natural eliminated in the body. If someone is having cancer grow then their body is toxic and their sewage system is backed up. Just like a real life sewage facility. If it backed up and started spewing toxic waste out of its "pores" pipes and gutters. Then the town would get sick. So would does your body. Now in the next chapter we will target specific parts of the body like the kidneys and liver and go into what best detox's them. Now for overall detoxing. You have got to eat clean, limit your intake of sugar. Limit all junk food, no dairy products, no yeast, eat clean like your great ancestors did. Pure food for a pure body. Lots of greens and vegetables. Get them minerals and vitamins into your body so your immune system can build up and heal itself, and detox the toxins. Juicing is great, I will recommend "liferegenerator" on YouTube. He has a great channel about raw/clean eating and living. He is very knowable and knows what he is doing. Exercising is great. It pumps up your heart and works your lungs so they may get bigger and more beneficial and filter your body more. When you sweat, toxins come out of your body. The inside comes out. That why sweating people smell bad. All the toxins come out. It has been noted that people who eat clean, raw diets and have great health give off little to no odor when they sweat. For they have little to no toxins. Why most people's pee and waste smell. Because of all the toxins and chemicals oozing out. Sleep is good. Good for your body, mind, spirit and mood! Beauty sleep is real. When you sleep your body recovers, heals and replenishes. Like an army resting after a fight and gets ready to fight another day. Basically you got to get your PH level up, eat clean food, exercise and get great sleep. Its basically chemistry, its natural and it works.

*Note When you detox, prepare for withdraws, sugar is a drug. So is coffee. And with most drugs, you get withdraws. All the toxins and chemicals that have been building up in your body over the years now must come out. Like a dictator that oppresses his people and doesn't want to leave. So will be the toxins, chemicals and parasites in your body. Better sooner than later. Detoxing is a great thing. It clears out the toxins and clears the mind more. For a buildup of toxins can clog the brain and its abilities. When you're detoxing eat slowly and chew your food well. The goal is to reduce the amount of work your digestive system has to do so it make clean itself out. Reduce your meat intake while detoxing will definitely help the body for meat takes a long time to digest for it is heavier in protein. Fruits are great, and they do the body much good with their vitamins and nutrients. Just don't over eat them, for they still contain sugar, not as much as a coke or as bad as Twinkies but you want to keep your sugar levels down. Cancer eats sugar. Eating lots of greens and colorful variety of vegetables daily is a great way to combat cancer. Getting raw garlic and cutting it up is fantastic for the body and immune system, garlic is loaded with sulfur that just eradicates toxins and is wonderful for cleaning out the blood stream. Avocados and grapefruit are rich in glutathione which the Huffington post had called "The Mother of all antioxidants" antioxidants wage war on toxins

!!! A huge theory is that smoking weed cures cancer. I will tell you the truth. HELL NO IT DOSNT. Putting more toxins in your body will not rid your body of toxins. If weed cured cancer then Bob Marley would have not off died of cancer !!! Check mate pro pot people. Again it comes back to basic chemistry, alkaline and acidic. Why do government push to legalize weed ? So they can keep the people poor and stupid while robbing them with the enormous amounts of money they make off of legalization.

Many researches including BBC and CBS NEWS have shown that marijuana smoking has more toxins than cigarettes !!! Seen chapter 9 for article headline !!!

Cutting out dairy and peanut butter is crucial to helping the gut. I would go as far to say that Dairy is the #1 cause of gut problems and acne !!! Switching to almond milk is a far better alternative.

Chapter 6 : Detoxing The Gut!

Your gut is your health. Where the majority of your immune system is. Healthy gut, healthy body. Your gut contain a lot of bacteria. Despite what you may have heard. Not all bacteria is bad. Your gut has good bacteria (Gut Flora) and then the bad bacteria. Gut Flora helps digest the food and break it down. Not having enough can lead to weak stomach acid and many sicknesses and diseases. When your gut flora is low. Foreign invades can move in and dominate your gut. Such a yeast for example. Without good gut flora to balance out your stomach yeast can rise and start an infection. Yeast can toxify the body in the majority for it latches on to the stomach and makes holes in your stomach. This can cause people to feel sick right after eating. Multitudes of people have yeast infections. They suffer in different ways. Yeast, like cancer and many other foreign invaders eat sugar and grow rapidly in a toxic, acidic sugary environment. Now to get that gut flora back in control. Lots of water, cutting up raw garlic and digesting it helps defeat the yeast. Drinking apple cider vinegar helps the stomach acid and is recommend using before and after meals if you have low acid levels in your gut. It has been noted that some people have even cured acne with ACV (Apple Cider Vinegar) Squeezing lemons and limes into water is well known for detoxing the body. Some signs of having bad gut health are: You get sick a lot. You get sick easily. Being overweight, bloating, constipation, fatigue, acne, diabetes, trouble losing weight. Not using the bathroom regularly. Putting magnesium powder in your water is great way to clean your bowls and get them moving.

*Warning: This will clean your system. It really will. Use it when you have a period of free time because your bowls will move after taking it and you will use the restroom. Also to be noted. Do not take to much magnesium.

What is great for your stomach is to have it do as little work as possible. If you cook your food, cook it well. Avoid red meat. Chew well, for digestion begins in the mouth. The less work your stomach does, the better. For the less work it does, the less energy it consumes and the less stress it goes through. For a tired stressed out stomach is ripe for toxins and diseases like a tired person and a trap. Eating fiber rich foods helps move the bowls and has been proven to reduce colon cancer. You don't want anything to stay to long in your digestive track. For when food remains in your stomach too long. Bad bacteria and toxins can multiply more and your stomach is occupied with digesting and can not divert full attention to the bad bacteria and such. Eating a lot of vegetables and a few fruits is great for cleaning the stomach. Its natural food for your natural body. Plus they are full of vitamins, fiber and other great stuff that does wonders in your body. Eating raw foods (Not Meat) is food in its natural state which is easier for the stomach to process.

*Note : You may lose weight once you clean your stomach/bowels by doing what is recommended on the last few pages. Also it will be easier to lose weight for your stomach and bowels are clean and can process foods better. Also you may get headaches and fell tired for your body is doing a mass, much needed deportation of chemicals and toxins. This will consume a good amount of your body's energy and will stress the organs. It is better to do this sooner than later. Drink lots of water during this process to better flush the toxins out. My mother juiced for a week and went running. She lost 15 pounds in one week !!!

Chapter 7 : Detoxing The Liver !!

When the liver is overworked. It cannot deport toxins and fats a maximum output. A lot of alcohol and drugs get sent to the liver and they do a lot of damage. Once your liver is fully clean, you may drink alcohol conservatively. But during detox, please refrain from consuming alcohol and taking pills. For it is hard to keep a house clean when someone is always behind you messing up what you clean. So is consuming junk food/alcohol/pills during detoxing. Detoxing can take a lot of the body, so if it your first time, you may feel rough. There are many food that assist the Liver in flushing out toxins. Consuming a small amount of raw garlic triggers the release of enzymes which helps the body break down food and flush out toxins. Grapefruit is high in Vitamin C and antioxidants which has the natural cleansing ability to clean the liver. Raw or juiced beats and carrots contain great amount of vitamins that improve overall liver function. Carrots are also great for your eyesight ! One of the most biggest and widely used items for enjoyment and detoxing is mostly overlooked. That is great for all detoxing is green tea. Full of plant antioxidants that assist the liver. Green vegetables are powerful for the body, their alkaline, contain tons of vitamins, flowing with plant chlorophyll that are like trees in the body, soaking up all the toxins and chemical particles floating around. That is how you detox the Liver !!!

Chapter 8 : Detoxing The Kidneys !!!

The kidneys are very important in the body's sewage system. They filter out toxins and help with the body's circulation. Consuming foods and drinks that are high in antioxidants and electrolytes will help. Consuming electrolytes will give your body energy. A kidney cleanse is great for those with kidney problems such as kidney stone. Limiting sugar is a must, if you're going to eat sugar let it be natural sugar from fruits not processed foods. Certainly not anything out of a can. Coconut juice is great for detoxing. Drinking a lot of it will certainly flush your system and move your bowels. Some super rich antioxidant fruits are cranberries, black cherries and blueberries. Drinking cranberry juice will detox the kidneys. Just do over do it on the fruit, cause remember...... You got to watch and limit your sugar intake. If you're going to be juicing, juicing cranberries and celery will do it. Adding beats to your juice will work your body wonders in detoxing the kidneys and beats are great for cleansing the blood. Drinking green tea will also help. If you want to try something new. Seaweed and kelp will clean you out. So will squeezing raw lemons and lime into your water. Grapes are tasty, they are also a great source of potassium. Ginger root and Turmeric are champions in detoxing. Both of them do wonders in the body and for detoxing. Drinking tea or apple cider vinegar before and after a meal will help the digestive system process its contains faster and more effective. Now if you're going to juice. Buy natural/organic fruits and vegetables. They are cheap to buy and will not include the deadly pesticides and cancer causing chemicals on non-organic fruits and vegetables.

Chapter 9: News Articles Connecting Food To Cancer !

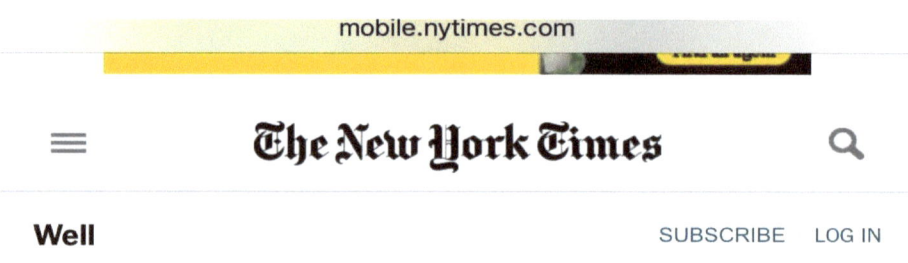

Can Foods Affect Colon Cancer Survival?

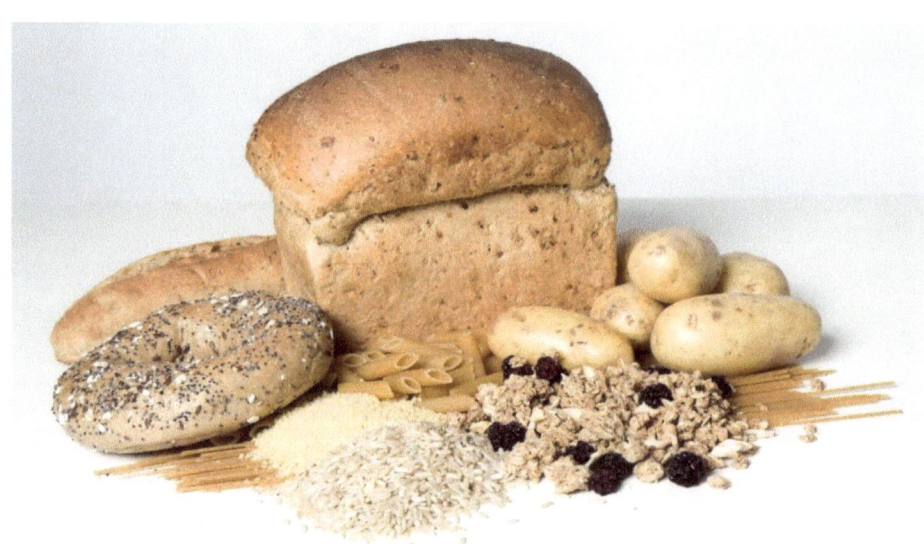

Whole-grain foods and others with a low glycemic load may protect against colon cancer recurrence.

By ANAHAD O'CONNOR
NOVEMBER 9, 2012

A new study suggests that what you eat may affect your chances of surviving colon cancer.

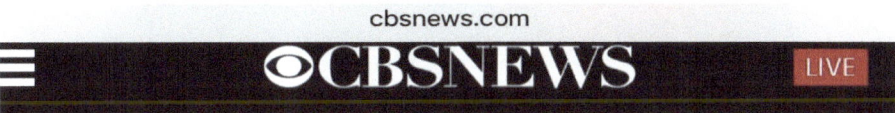

Health: WebMD

Study Shows Toxins in Marijuana Smoke

 WEBMD
Dec 17, 2007 4:30 PM EST

New research from Canada shows that some toxins may be more
abundant in marijuana cigarettes than tobacco cigarettes.

The researchers burned 30 marijuana cigarettes and 30 tobacco cigarettes on
a machine in their lab, measuring levels of chemicals in the smoke.

Ammonia levels were up to 20 times higher in marijuana smoke than in tobacco
smoke. Levels of hydrogen cyanide and nitrogen-related chemicals were
three to five times higher in marijuana smoke than in tobacco smoke.

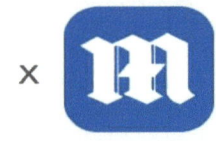
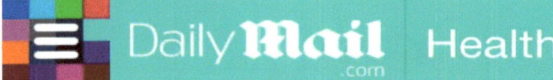

Daily **Mail** Health

...now believe that the link between dairy produce and breast cancer is similar to the link between smoking and lung cancer. It was difficult to accept that a substance as "natural" as milk might have such ominous health implications, but I am living proof that it worked.

Cutting out dairy produce is one of the main dietary points, but there are other very important ones. You should eat masses of vege- tables and fruit (with more emph- asis on vegetables) - not only are they full of vitamins, minerals and antioxidants, but many contain chemicals which have anticancer properties, such as allicin in garlic, or lycopene in tomatoes. You should limit your intake of saturated fats, and eat a diet rich in monounsaturates (such as olive oil), and omega 3 and 6 oils (oily fish, flax seeds and nuts). Eating adequate amounts of protein is important for your body - though I suggest that as much as possible should be from vegetable sources (eg, lentils); salt and sugar should be kept to a minimum, in favour of seasonings which have anti-cancer action, such as the curcumin in turmeric.

Genetically Modified Foods (GMOs) and Cancer

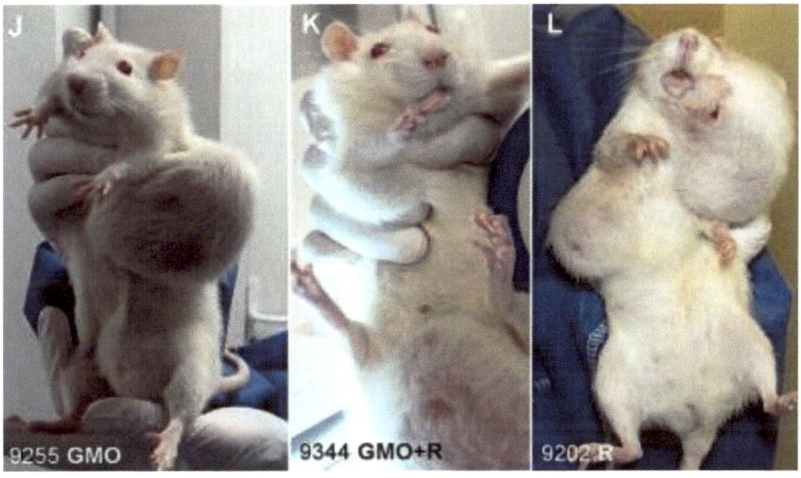

A recent peer-reviewed study (published in the Food and Chemical Toxicology Journal) has linked genetically modified foods to an increase in cancer risk in laboratory animals. In the study, the rats fed on genetically modified corn died prematurely, many of which having tumours the size of golf balls. 50% of the males and 70% of the females died prematurely as a result of a GMO diet. Not only did these rats have tumours, they

▶ Watch **One-Minute World News**

Last Updated: Wednesday, 19 December 2007, 01:0

✉ E-mail this to a friend   🖨 Printable version

Cannabis smoke 'has more toxins'

Inhaled cannabis smoke has more harmful toxins than tobacco, scientists have discovered.

The Canadian government research found 20 times as much ammonia, a chemical linked to cancer, New Scientist said.

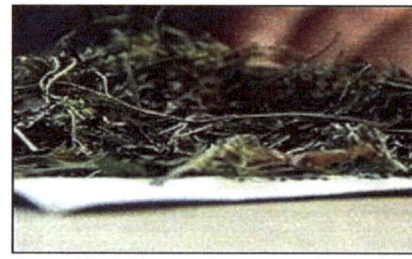

Cannabis is the most commonly used illegal drug

The Health Canada team also found five times as much hydrogen cyanide and nitrogen oxides, which are linked to heart and lung damage respectively.

But tobacco smoke contained more of a toxin linked to infertility. Experts said users must be aware of the risks.

About a quarter of the population in the UK smokes tobacco products, while a sixth of 15 to 34-year-olds have tried cannabis in the past year, making it the most commonly used drug.

Previous research has shown cannabis smoke is more harmful to lungs than tobacco as it is inhaled more deeply and held in the lungs for a longer period.

> 66 **The confirmation of the presence of known carcinogens and other chemicals implicated is important information for public health** 99
>
> David Moir, lead researcher

However, it has also been acknowledged that the average tobacco user smokes more than a cannabis user.

Researchers from Health Canada, the government's

SEE ALS
▸ Cannab
31 Jul (
▸ Cannab
27 Jul (
▸ Cannab
18 Jul (
▸ Judge v
19 Jul (
▸ 'My lun
repair'
03 Jun

RELATED
▸ British
▸ New Sc
▸ Health
The BBC
content (

TOP HEA
▸ Stem c
▸ Hospita
▸ Low vit
🔊 | N

MOST PC

MOST S
1 BBC
2 Ted (
   race
3 BBC
4 US e
   resul
5 BBC
6 BBC
7 BBC
8 BBC
9 Sixtie

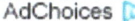

THE BLOG

A Cure For Cancer? Eating A Plant-Based Diet

🕐 Nov 24, 2009 | **Updated** Nov 17, 2011

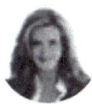

Kathy Freston Health and Wellness Activist, Author

I have been working closely recently with a few extraordinary nutritional researchers, and I find that the information they have compiled is quite eye opening. Interestingly, what these highly esteemed doctors are saying is just beginning to be understood and accepted, perhaps because what they are saying does not conveniently fit in with or support the multi-billion dollar food industries that profit from our "not knowing". One thing is for sure: we are getting sicker and more obese than our health care system can handle, and the conventional methods of dealing with disease often have harmful side effects and are ineffective for some patients.

     +

Chapter 10: About The Author

Conor A. Murphy is a young man from San Diego California. Son of Eileen Murphy from Waterford Ireland. While attending school. Mr. Murphy ate a lot of processed, high sugar, gmo and dairy junk food. His gut was wreaked and he had many illnesses and got sick quite often from his eating habits. His knowledgeable mother lead him to a "clean living" and thus begin a spark inside his brain where eating good, quality, nutritious food became a way of life and he has never, been in such good health. He rarely get sick, and he no longer feels sick after eating food. All thanks to his wonderful God given Mother. Thank You Mother !!!

*This book is volume #1 in a new series called " True Health " which will inform the masses about the truth health of the body, understanding how the body works, what benefits and helps the body, and what harms the body. Very interesting, and COMING SOON !!!